My little pillow book...

I take everywhere

Laura Melguizo Pérez

For A, IA, the ginger haired
and all who came here
before us.

What makes me happy

Snow, white, silent, halting the dullness of
the day; it makes me be a little one again.

Colour green, as emeralds are, as Ireland
is, like trees when first leafs are just buds
in spring and moss is covered of dew
drops.

White round pebbles like small eggs, and
black and flat pebbles like vinyl records,
all soft and polished, when you find them
while taking a walk on the countryside.

Swifts, swallows and house martins, when
they stop for some days to hunt and take
a rest on their migration. Cranes, geese,
with their shouts. The enormous starling
murmurations, that hypnotize with their
almost impossible choreography.

Those few movies where you get into them so deep that you live each moment as part of the cast and suffer for not being able to be listened by the main character but, at the end, whatever it is, you feel relief of what happened. That cathartic experience so exhausting but... what a joy.

Red and white irish setters. Furry, crazy, charming, soft and clever. Knowing a thousand games, always taking your hand where they love to be scratched. They are just happy, just because.

Rain on the window, happy, sad, monotonal, without rhythm, windy or not. Relaxing.

The Storm, it comes, and it leaves. With its scandal, its music, its strength, its light, its submission, its ability to bring fear, pain. The scent and suspense when it

comes; the clear air, fresh, and the
calmed spirit, when it leaves.

The indescribable moments, that are pure
happiness, but that are secret ones, and
you keep them for the harsh moments, to
soothe them, and regain strength.

Spend hours talking about everything and
nothing, with that person who you don't
need to say a word so he knows exactly
what you means or, simply, to share
silence on good company.

Come upon a tale, story, place, painting or
song that brings me a message or idea I
have never thought of or could never
come across my mind, and it pleases mes.

Fear

Many times I have fear. Some times I forget that fear is something natural that allows me to survive.

I know fear is part of me, but some times, it doesn't let me see around me, and don't find an exit. It won't go away, but it'll become smaller and then it'll allow me to find a path to follow.

Those called the brave ones, in fact they had fear too; those who took the risk and won or lost everything, also had that moment where fear clouds the senses and don't let continue. And despite everything, they made the fear smaller, and with it beside them, carry on.

I have decided to befriend fear, because it alerts me when risks are close, my survival can depend on it, and I'm grateful for this primal instinct that lets me be in contact with nature itself.

Also, I'm going to be a good friend of my fear, I won't feed it, but I want to listen to it when it speaks and enjoy its company, as it will be always by mi side.

When I'm with those other persons who speaks about their fears and experiences with it, I always learn something new to talk with mine. It's nice to know strategies of others when own doesn't seem to work, so trying those others.

Autumn

Three Doors, poem from Chinato, sang by
Robe[1]. Violins and Electric Guitars.

Leaves changing colours, flying and
dancing, oranges, reddle, terracotta,
ochre, red, brown; rainbow of heat that
falls to the ground.

Rain returns, but less that langsyne, as
they say. Grey days, breeze days, they are
the smile of Moncayo mountain calling
the first frosts at the end of November.

North wind blows with the intend to make
us remember it is the Lord of the valley,
and that comes from our ancestors lands,
and he brings messages from the ones
who departed.

[1]   These are related to a song called "Tres
puertas" from Estrechinato y Tu, lyrics from the poet
known as Chinato.

It's already very noticeable how short
days are, last night so early, sun forgets to
get up early. I'm always sleepy.

Weather is so changing, just like my
mood. I don't know if I'm sad because it
rains, or it rains because I'm sad; I only
know that today I'm sad and it's raining,
and yesterday was raining and I was
happy.

I would like to think that with all this rain
air is purified and we can breath better,
but people are stubborn taking their cars;
run and get busy trying not to get soaked,
and I read a quote about this matter from
the Hagakure.

There are holidays for every like, noise,
noise and more noise; but, over all, mobs
of people who crowd and jostle for the
"free" word and the noise by pleasure of
noise, and the untempered speakers to be

heard so high and so far. Spending for spending, and it was before a matter of praying.

There they are, pumpkins, soups, scent to roasted chestnut and churrería[2]. I'd like an italian ice cream but it's closed because people don't attend it, what a pity, it's so scrumptious that almost hand made venetian straciatella. Grazie mille, Aldo.

Again I'm thinking of leaves, how they turn into caramel colour, like setter, red and white; roasted apples, experiments making a fire with pine cones and twigs and get warm with that crackling and happy music. Outside, chimney's smoke melt with the shreds of fog, stubborn on staying.

---

[2]   Typical season shop that serves a fried pastry called churro.

Winter

You are the dream of the snow, dull days
and nights, expecting the white shine of
the still clouds.

Drawing smiling faces on the glass;
messages on the blurred windows of the
city bus to make happy an unknown
passenger I will never met.

Smell of fire, quiet nature, fleeing people,
thinking this is the death season.

The first ray of light the next day of
solstice, a bit sooner, the last, a second
later. More light hours, What is waiting
nature, so still and like sleeping? It may be
that, with cold, it prefers like me to
snuggle, and sleep and share love and
warmness with the closest ones.

I see people, at the days when it all starts, willing to spend as there was no tomorrow, spend money, things, visits, calls, cards, food, and much more; do they remember the scent of the roasted chestnut women on the avenue? Festive lights? Clouds and the first snowflakes falling down?

Many times they say that my behaviour is as a little girl waiting to know snow for the first time. Naive, as simple-hearted as a bucket upside down, they say. I do prefer to be innocent, so, I will always will find wonder on little things that make life really worthy.

I like winter, it's like a mother waiting a new being inside her, or the embers of fire, in the morning, that looks like the bonfire is extinct but, if you throw some twigs, and tell how much you love him, it flares again and warms home.

Silence

So little things so worthy as silence is. We live surrounded by noise, I wonder what reasons push us to torture ourselves so eagerly with it. It's so deafening and painfully that most of the time I need to block it.

Pure silence can also be terrifying; as human mind works, searching for sounds, something, as own blood flowing. It's like going out to the streets early in a sunday morning and not listening to a car on the empty roads, but the birds, a happy dog barking because it's about to take a walk outside.

It's a park full of kids, without phones, or video game consoles, just playing and having fun. It's the forest, the park, the grove, mutter of animals playing peek-a-boo.

It's the meteor shower, rain or snow in the middle of the nigh, soft and silent melody of dreams, magic and quietness. It's the old lore cave where our ancestor lived, the temple where we pray, the top of the mountain and the walls where the sea waves break. It's closing your eyes and just feeling how breathing works.

If people chose silence more frequently, would realize how easy it is to concentrate when noise is not around, thinking happen, listening to the thoughts, knowing self better.

Wind

I must confess that when it blows hard
some days in a row, it gives me a
headache, but at least it takes pollution in
suspension away from the city.

Sometimes it blows so strong that the
blind down and windows closed they
shakes a lot, they seem to be blown away
at any time. When I was younger it scared
me, so much to have nightmares; one day
I thought it would be great that, if blind
and windows were blown away, the air
stream could take me just like Dorothy, to
the Land of Oz.

Some other times, when it blows so
smooth, I try to listen to its voice, like a
whisper, as Capote told us, but not only
from the ones who left us, also the ones
who are far and love us and we love too.

I always think it's a living being, in fact, because it's unpredictable, going back and forth, as it pleases, when he likes, with the power it will. Sometimes he is your companion, others it pushes you to your destiny, others it push you way to avoid you suffering and others, it exploded with joy when it mixes with rain and fire, while the best storms.

It's a brave gentleman, who bring us the perfume of surrounding plants, no matter they are out of the city, from fire, water, storm, snow and fog. Scent to rosemary, thyme and lavender.

Wind, when I feel the longing of that I cannot describe or understand where it comes from, as it's deep and primal, carry me into your arms to find the answers of that call from the wild.

Wealth and Money

Money: coins, bills, plastic cards. That's not wealth, it's only a way to fulfill basic needs. It won't make me happy, but will ease my mind that it helps me avoiding worse problems. Wealth is other thing, it's what makes me feel full, joyful, dreamy, complete. A good book, a chat, a glance and a song hummed by a little kid while playing and day dreaming.

Sometimes I feel poor, really poor, with the need to look for a corner on any street and, with the crying in the words, mumble to the passersby: alms, an alm[3]!

Other times I feel so overflowing of wealth, so plentiful, that hugs fall from my pockets, songs and music scatter as the

---

[3] Pun made with the spanish world "alma", meaning soul. Has the same intention in spanish version.

day was a musical and people had forgotten their character on the play, and run to avoid appearing in the rehearsals; and it's so merry to sing out of tune all together and miss the show...

In fact, we don't know the value of money, if it has any. Some people say it's the value banks give it, or market or, as they say at home, the effort it takes to earn it. As anyone seems to agree, I have decided that money is a living being to care and treat respectful and lovingly, and giving it the chance to be part of my life, with no judgment, and give it space and time and dedication to grow, like any other plant or animal.

I have seen some persons who had lot of money but were very poor, and vice versa. I feel lucky for knowing how to pick out money and wealth, even when I'm so sad I feel poor, I know money won't make me rich again, but a bit of happiness.

Music

I always have a song in my mind. No matter if I'm listening to it through the air, or just playing it in my head.

When there is no sound but the melody in my mind, this is a kind of silence that fills and relaxes mes. It's my favorite radio station, I always listen live those amazing players and conductors who are not here with us anymore.

I like written music, it's like a mathematical equation with an amazing result. They may say that the best musicians are great mathematicians, but they don't like to hear this comment; however, they have revealed the music of spheres.

I like children and animals reactions to classical music, because is unveils their sensibility, their soul. Music is a universal language, it doesn't need the convention of words or gestures that we were taught in our culture, it allows us to understand anyway.

Sometimes I would love that life were more like a musical. It would be fun and quaint that, suddenly, you were into a story that has nothing to do with you, singing and dancing, and you are that kind of person who always say that cannot dance two steps without stomp others feet or detune is singing better than you, but there you are. I believe we would be happier and would have less fear of ridicule, we would be less conditioned.

And if I want to sing, I do sing, and I want to dance, and I do it really bad, I dance, and if I want to hear the ninth of Mahler, well, then I think you better come and hug me and suggest me something from Mozart for little children.

If I could ask to learn playing an instrument, I would learn playing piano or violin. They are that kind of beings that can transform a bit of ink in a sheet of paper the happiest into the most devastated crying one, or the miserable dance of joy. Maybe it's because they have a voice like ours, and can send the emotions from the composer who wrote the music sheet, from the player, the listener, even from the wood and herd each piece comes from.

Although there is some music out of my likes, all music is beautiful.